ARTHRITIS —
cause and control
(The Pantothenic Acid Theory)

E C Barton-Wright D Sc., FRIC, FI Biol.

ISBN 0 906202 04 3   Published by Bunterbird Limited

ARTHRITIS — CAUSE AND CONTROL

First published 1975
Second Edition 1978
Third Edition 1982

© Dr. E C Barton Wright 1975

Formerly published by Roberts Publications
as 'Arthritis its Cause and Control' with the
ISBN 0 906185 04 1. Now published with
additions by:

Bunterbird Ltd
225 Putney Bridge Road
London SW15 2PY England

ISBN 0 906202 04 3

Printed in Great Britain by Errand Press, Portsmouth

Contents

Introduction

This booklet has been specially written for the layman who is assumed to have little or no knowledge of biochemistry, in as simple and non-technical language as possible, and is about the author's views on the cause and prevention of that crippling disease, arthritis, which is increasing at the present time at an alarming rate in nearly every country in the world.

The author's basic contention is that arthritis, using the term to include its many and wide manifestations, is a vitamin deficiency disease caused by the consumption in our daily diet of inadequate amounts of the vitamin "pantothenic acid", a member of the B-complex, over many years.

For the layman I would first like to define what a vitamin is. It has been known for many years that in addition to proteins, fats, carbohydrates, mineral salts and water, a perfect diet must include a number of relatively simple natural organic substances to maintain the complete health and well-being of animals. The daily requirements of these substances by different species and individuals varies enormously and the actual amounts required are small compared with the bulk of the daily diet consumed, but tiny though these amounts are, they are vitally necessary for the normal growth and health of an animal. If certain specific vitamins are completely absent in the diet, which is rare, or present in inadequate amounts, "deficiency diseases", such as scurvy, beri-beri, pellagra and rickets make their appearance.

These substances are each unique and perfectly specific in their biological functions and cannot replace one another in our diet. Moreover, they must *all* be present in adequate amounts if perfect health is to be maintained. With one possible exception (vitamin D), these compounds must be supplied in our food and they are collectively known as *"vitamins"*, because the body cannot make them for itself.

Vitamins have been divided into two classes: "fat-soluble" and "water-soluble". They were originally labelled alphabetically; A, B, C, D, E, etc., but "vitamin B" proved to be a complex mixture of unique water-soluble substances and is now termed the vitamin B-complex.

Arthritis is defined as a disease of the joints and the name is derived from two Greek words; *arthron*, joint and the suffix *itis*, inflammation: in other words a disease characterized by the inflammation of the joints. It has two principal forms; *rheumatoid* and *osteoarthritis*.

As a rule rheumatoid arthritis attacks women more than men; the proportion being about 7 women to 1 man, and the disease most commonly appears in females between the ages of 20 and 40. Rheumatoid arthritis usually attacks the extremities of the body, i.e., hands and feet, and in very advanced cases the shoulders, and is accompanied by varying degrees of crippling joint deformities associated with the inflammation and wastage of muscle tissue round the affected joints and its severity increases with time. Osteoarthritis, as the name implies (Gr. *osteon*, bone, *arthron*, joint and *itis*, inflammation) is a disease affecting the bony structures of the body. It may be a primary condition, or may follow injury, such as a violent blow, or fracture of a bone (traumatic arthritis); this is a very common form of arthritis among race horses. In a joint, the ends of the bones are covered by a smooth self-lubricating substance called *cartilage* and the whole joint is contained in a capsule of fibrous tissue attached to both bones and lined by the thin *synovial membrane* which contains the *synovial fluid*. In severe cases of osteoarthritis, the synovial membrane becomes worn and may even be entirely destroyed with the result that the joints actually grind against one another. There is also joint distortion caused by bony outgrowths or spurs (osteophytes) and general thickening of bone from compression or new formation.

Osteoarthritis can strike a number of different parts of the body i.e., hands, feet, knees, spine and shoulders. Osteoarthritis, unlike the rheumatoid form, affects more men than women and is also the commoner form of the disease and osteoarthritics outnumber rheumatoids by approximately 20 : 1.

Another form of arthritis that may be mentioned here is gout, which is a metabolic disorder in which sodium biurate (a uric acid compound), is deposited in the cartilages of the joints, as well as other parts of the body, for instance the ears. As a rule the big toe is involved and becomes swollen and extremely painful. The incidence of gout is generally ascribed to the consumption of large amounts of alcohol, especially port. This, however, is not altogether true, because teetotallers are also prone to gout. The disease is said to respond to treatment with panthothenic acid.

Yet another type of arthritis, at least in its early stages, is Still's disease. The disease was first described by the English physician, George Still (1868-1947). It is comparatively rare and usually attacks children between the ages of 3 and 6 years. Still's disease is a form of rheumatoid polyarthritis and unless it is thrown off naturally by the time puberty is reached, the child becomes a hopeless cripple for life.

Osteoporosis is a form of arthritis. Our bones are mainly constructed of the mineral salt calcium phosphate which gives them their rigidity. When a person suffers from osteoporosis, the calcium is leached out of the bones, which in consequence crumble and the patient is left in very great pain and in advanced states of the disease is virtually unable to walk.

An interesting case of osteoarthritis, which strongly supports the arguments to be given later, that arthritis is mainly a vitamin deficiency disease, comes from Russia. In a certain province of that country osteoarthritis is endemic, which means that a certain disease, in this case osteoarthritis, is peculiar to a region or group of people. A large proportion of the population living in this area suffer from softening of the ends of bones, thickening of the bones and ankylosis (stiffness or fixation of a joint). In other words, they have all the symptoms of severe osteoarthritis. It would be interesting to know the composition of the diet eaten by these people, but unfortunately I have not been able to obtain any information on this subject, but I am

3

willing to offer very long odds that their daily diet is woefully deficient in pantothenic acid.

Up to the present time the cause and control of any form of arthritis, with the exception of gout, where at any rate the cause is known, appears to have completely baffled the medical profession. Over 50 years ago it was suggested that rheumatoid arthritis was due to some kind of bacterial infection. This theory has recently been revived and large sums of money have been expended to discover and isolate this mysterious, elusive and in my opinion mythical organism. This is all very reminiscent of the early history of two notorious vitamin deficiency diseases; beri-beri or polyneuritis, and pellagra. After many years of painstaking research it was shown conclusively that neither beri-beri nor pellagra were bacterial diseases but were caused by inadequate amounts of two vitamins being consumed in the daily diet, namely vitamin B_1 (thiamine) for preventing beri-beri, and nicotinamide (niacinamide) for the prevention of pellagra. In both cases the medical profession conducted a vigorous and not very scrupulous campaign against the view that these really appalling diseases could be due to the deficiency of some specific factor in the diet and did not hesitate to persecute and ridicule the early pioneers in this field of nutrition.

What are the present views of the medical profession about the cause, much less the control or cure of the different forms of arthritis? The bacterial infection theory has already been mentioned. Another and more recent view, that seemingly has found much favour among those members of the medical profession specializing in this branch of medicine, is that arthritis is an auto-immune disease, which means that certain body tissues suddenly become treated by the defensive body mechanism as if they were foreign bodies, thus provoking an inflammatory condition. The evidence advanced for this theory appears to be as meagre as the bacterial infection theory and is based on no kind of scientific data whatsoever.

The question naturally arises here, what hope can the medical profession offer to sufferers from any form of arthritis? It is shocking to have to admit that after years of research and the expenditure of vast amounts of money, that the medical profession is just as ignorant today as it was a hundred years ago about the cause or causes of this crippling and extremely painful group of diseases, much less knowing how to cure or even control them.

The principal methods of treatment now in vogue are mere palliatives, which bring in their train a number of distressing and often disastrous side effects, and when these palliatives fail, as they invariably do, and the sufferer is in a far worse state than before treatment, he or she is told the not very comforting news: "Well, you must learn to live with the disease."

Analgesics, pain killers, and anti-inflammatory drugs have been much recommended and used, such as different forms of aspirin, phenylbutazone, indomethacin and cortisone. Only one of these substances is formed in our bodies, cortisone, all the others are synthetic laboratory products. They *all*, including cortisone, produce serious side effects, such as internal bleeding, oedema, nausea, rashes, reactivation of latent peptic ulcers, dizziness, headaches and many others.

Yet another method of treatment, which was all the fashion some years ago and afterwards abandoned because of its very serious side effects has recently been revived and that is the injection of gold in the form of a soluble compound. It is hard to understand why this treatment has been revived by intelligent and responsible men and women, who must be fully aware of its many and serious side effects, such as: dermatitis, hepatitis, stomatitis and nephritis which sometimes result in death.

Another type of injection treatment, which seems to be even more dangerous than gold therapy has been tried out in Mexico. It should be mentioned here that this treatment has been banned in the U.S.A. and presumably in Great Britain. The treatment consists in the injection of the powerful poison known by its initials, DMSO (dimethyl sulphoxide). DMSO is a poison in its own right and on contact with the skin can produce violent itching, while volunteers have reported: nausea, vomiting, cramps, chills, drowsiness following upon skin absorption and heavy bleeding from the nose and ears. Death has also been reported after this treatment. Nevertheless, in spite of these shocking side effects, this treatment is still being administered in Mexico, and apparently there is no lack of wealthy American patients who are willing to pay large fees and risk their lives by having it.

All forms of arthritis are extremely painful diseases, especially in the advanced state. It is little wonder, therefore, that sufferers will turn to any drug which will alleviate their agony, even if it be for a few hours, whatever may be the side effects. If, as the present author contends, the arthritic syndrome as it is called, is caused by eating a diet deficient in the vitamin pantothenic acid, pain killers and their relatives can at best merely relieve the pain for a short time, but unfortunately with the recurrence of the symptoms, patients come more and more to rely upon these pain killers, even if they only serve to alleviate their misery temporarily.

It is idle to tell arthritic sufferers that prevention is better than cure and that they should have seen to it that they consumed a daily diet containing adequate amounts of pantothenic acid, even from early infancy, since once a person has become afflicted with any form of arthritis, it is, unlike other vitamin deficiency diseases, extremely difficult to control. In fact, in the vast majority of cases there is no permanent cure, any more than there is a permanent cure for diabetes. Diabetes, however, can be controlled by keeping to a strict dietary schedule coupled with daily injections of the pancreatic hormone insulin. In such circumstances the diabetic can lead a long and useful life. In the same way it is hoped to show later in this booklet that arthritics can also lead a pain-free existence if the treatment to be described is strictly followed.

What is Pantothenic Acid?

In 1933 Dr. Roger J. Williams of Texas University, Austen, Texas, U.S.A. found a substance to be present in an aqueous extract of rice husks that was capable of stimulating the growth of various bacteria and yeasts to a remarkable degree. From its apparently universal distribution in the plant and animal world, Williams instead of calling it vitamin B_5, as he should have done, named it "pantothenic acid", from the Greek word *pantothen* meaning *from everywhere*.

Williams and his collaborators showed that pantothenic acid is a pale yellow, rather viscous oily substance. The acid itself was fairly unstable, but the calcium salt was found to be relatively stable and is the form in which pantothenic acid is available to the public.

Although pantothenic acid is widely distributed in all the foods we eat, the amounts available are, with certain exceptions, very small. The richest sources of the acid as far as our food is concerned are: liver, rice husks, egg yolks, royal jelly, cod ovaries, soybeans, dried peas, peanuts and brewers' yeasts.

Pantothenic acid is absorbed through the intestines and since it is water-soluble it is excreted in urine and sweat. Although the vast bulk of our intake of pantothenic acid is from the food we eat, nevertheless, there is a small amount synthesized by our intestinal bacterial flora; a fact which may partly account for the slow onset of arthritis.

It was soon realised that pantothenic acid itself is not the functional form of the vitamin in the body and it was shown nearly 30 years ago that it formed part of an important enzyme system known as coenzyme A, which is concerned with the oxidation of sugars in our bodies by means of the so-called Krebs cycle. Not only does pantothenic acid form an integral part of coenzyme A, but it also controls the formation of the cortico-steroid hormones in our adrenal glands.

The adrenal glands in our bodies are two small glands which are situated on the upper surface of the kidneys and are composed of two different kinds of tissue. There is a small inner portion called the *medulla*, which is composed of tissue of the nervous type and secretes two hormones, adrenaline and noradrenaline, and a wide outer layer called the *cortex* consisting of glandular tissue. It is this adrenal cortex which is the seat of synthesis or production of these cortico-steroid hormones, such as, cortisone, aldosterone and some 30 others including the sex hormones.

Although the glands in our bodies have been known to anatomists for many hundreds of years, it is only within comparatively recent times that they have been recognised as organs which have the property of secreting chemical substances called *hormones* or *chemical messengers,* which are of great biological importance, into the blood stream. Those glands which secrete hormones directly into the blood stream are known as *ductless* or *endocrine* glands and sometimes as organs of internal secretion.

Hormones, like vitamins, are capable of carrying out physiological reactions in the body out of all proportion to their actual concentration. For example, it has been shown that the hormone adrenaline, which it will be remembered is formed in the adrenal medulla, is extremely active when present in the blood stream in a concentration of less than one part in one hundred million. Another feature of these ductless or endocrine glands is a plentiful blood supply that can carry these hormones rapidly to all parts of the body.

The adrenal cortex in mammals is extremely sensitive to dietary deficiencies. Lack of pantothenic acid, or sub-optimal amounts of the vitamin lead to atrophy (shrivelling up) of the cortical cells, which become filled with blood and many die, with the result that the cortico-steroid hormones, such as cortisone, are either not formed, or only in inadequate amounts, leading to symptoms of stress. Moreover, it only requires a very slight fall in the concentration of pantothenic acid to lead to significant falls in the production of these hormones.

The whole question of the relationship of pantothenic acid and the normal functioning of the adrenal glands is a very complicated one. There is, however, one important point that must be mentioned here, namely, if the adrenals are deprived of pantothenic acid over a long period of time, repair and recovery of the glandular tissues are slow and uncertain. This result, as will be seen later, may also play a part in the slow recovery of some arthritics with pantothenic acid treatment when the disease has been allowed to reach an advanced stage.

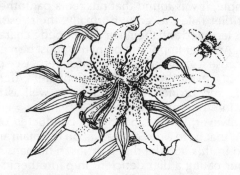

The Pantothenic Acid Requirements of Micro-Organisms and Insects

Pantothenic acid is an essential factor for the growth of many bacteria and yeasts. It is also an essential factor for the growth and development of many insects.

It is, however, "Royal Jelly", or Queen bee food, that is the classical example of pantothenic acid being essential to insects, because royal jelly has the remarkable property of converting any bee larva into a Queen. For many years it was considered that royal jelly contained the highest concentration of pantothenic acid of any natural product, but greater amounts have now been found in cod ovaries.

Effect of Pantothenic Acid Deficiency in Animals and Birds

The rat has probably been the most investigated animal as far as pantothenic acid deficiency in the diet is concerned. For example, it was found that rats fed a pantothenic acid deficient diet failed to grow normally, their resistance to stress was lessened and their hair developed a characteristic greyness. Another important point that must be mentioned here, because it arose in human "volunteers" (see below) is that rats fed a pantothenic acid deficient diet suffered from bronchitis and broncho-pneumonia, as well as hepatitis and fatty infiltration in the liver.

It is, however, some experiments conducted on rats in the U.S.A. that have a direct bearing on the main argument advanced in this booklet that arthritis in humans is chiefly due to our eating a diet deficient in pantothenic acid.

In this very important experiment, which appears to have been completely ignored by both nutritionists and the medical profession, freshly weaned rats were placed on a complete diet, but entirely lacking pantothenic acid. At the end of the experiment these rats showed all the symptoms of advanced osteoarthritis in their joints closely simulating osteoarthritis in humans.

Osteoarthritis in dogs, more especially among pedigree animals has been increasing during the last 10 to 15 years and is most probably due to these animals being mainly fed on highly processed canned foods. The author has noticed in his analyses conducted over the last 20 years of the vitamin content of different canned animal foods, a marked and significant fall in their pantothenic acid content. For example, 12 to 18 years ago the average pantothenic acid content of these canned foods was 4.5mg/lb. which is probably adequate to maintain the average weight dog in health. The value has now fallen to 1.2-1.5mg/lb, which might just suffice for toy types, but is grossly insufficient for bigger breeds. Some remarkable cures have been obtained in the U.S.A. by smearing a few milligrams of royal jelly on the tongues of dogs suffering from osteoarthritis plus 100mg of calcium pantothenate daily.

Pigs fed on a pantothenic acid deficient diet become extremely thin and emaciated and develop a rough coat with loss of hair. They suffer from diarrhoea and slow degenerative changes in their peripheral nerves. They also develop what has come to be called "goose-stepping gait" in their hind legs, i.e., there is lack of co-ordination in gait due to the development of osteoarthritis in their leg joints.

A deficiency of pantothenic acid in the diet of young chicks leads to extensive damage to the spinal cord, as well as causing dermatitis, fatty liver and retarded feathering. Drastic pantothenic acid deficiency in the food of breeder hens leads to a high loss of reproduction and hatchability of the eggs and it is now the custom to fortify the diet of breeder hens with calcium pantothenate.

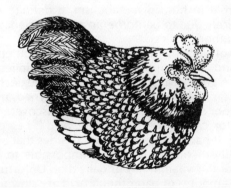

Pantothenic Acid Requirements of Humans

As recently as 1968 the Merck Index stated quite dogmatically that human requirements and deficiency syndrome of pantothenic acid had not yet been established, while the U.S.A. Federal Drug Administration (F.D.A.) at one time compelled manufacturers of calcium pantothenate to print on their labels: "Essential for human nutrition not yet proved." This has since been rescinded, but the F.D.A. has now shifted onto a very different and dangerous tack and is attempting to ban the sale of all vitamin supplements of whatever kind on the extraordinary grounds that adequate amounts for maintaining health are eaten in our daily diet.

In the Heinz Handbook of Nutrition there appears this astonishing statement: "The daily requirements of pantothenic acid (in humans) is about 10-15mg daily. This requirement is apparently easily satisfied, *even by poor diets* (author's italics) since this substance plays an important role in human metabolism, *a definite clinical disease entirely due to pantothenic acid deficiency is not known.*" (author's italics).

Instances of ignoring the importance of pantothenic acid in human and animal nutrition could be multiplied many times over. A great deal of the blame for the neglect of this vitamin, so far as human nutrition is concerned, must be laid at the door of Dr. Roger Williams, the discoverer of this substance, for calling it "pantothenic acid", i.e., present everywhere. It has been assumed on all sides that because of its ubiquitous distribution, it is impossible to have a deficiency of this vitamin in our daily diet. Unfortunately, inadequate amounts of pantothenic acid are slow to show their effects; especially as far as arthritis is concerned.

When the National Health Act was passed in 1947, and the Cohen Committee appointed to determine what drugs should or should not be prescribed under the Act, the Committee came to the conclusion that the following water-soluble vitamins were "musts": Thiamine, riboflavin, niacin and ascorbic acid, but when it came to the turn of pantothenic acid, it was vetoed on the grounds that since it was present in all foodstuffs there could not possibly be a lack of this vitamin in our daily diet; thereby blissfully ignoring the fact that the substance is fairly unstable and especially sensitive to dry heat and large amounts are destroyed in roasting, toasting and grilling. Pantothenic

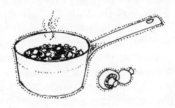

acid is also partially destroyed by pasteurization and even boiling. For example, it has been found that there is on the average a loss of 56% when such vegetables as Brussels sprouts, broccoli, spinach, mushrooms, tomatoes, etc., are canned. It was shown over 20 years ago that there is even a loss of pantothenic acid from defrosting frozen meat. Meats vary considerably in their susceptibility to heat destruction of pantothenic acid. For example, beef is particularly susceptible, even autoclaving for 15 minutes at 15 p.s.i. can cause 40-50% destruction of the vitamin, whereas mutton and pork appear to be unaffected. However, these experiments on mutton and pork do not show whether there might be considerable destruction of the vitamin when these substances are roasted or grilled.

Pantothenic acid is destroyed by some food preservatives. Milling of grains removes nearly 60% of the pantothenic acid and the fumigant methyl bromide, which is so widely used nowadays as an insecticide and rodenticide in silos and meat stores, entirely destroys pantothenic acid in the food fumigated, changing it into a new and totally useless substance.

Salicylic acid, formerly used as a food preservative, is known to destroy pantothenic acid. Since it is closely related to aspirin, it is possible that treatment of arthritis with aspirin could only eventually exacerbate the condition by destroying such pantothenic acid as may be present in the diet when it enters the intestinal tract.

It has also been stated that rancid fats destroy a number of vitamins, including pantothenic acid. Appreciable amounts of pantothenic acid may be lost in pan drippings in fried foods and the practice of serving gravies with meat and poultry may be a desirable practice.

Because bacterial flora in the intestine produce some pantothenic acid it must be remembered that use of antibiotics and antibacterial drugs in medicine kills much of this flora as well as the invading organisms. Thus, in any period of illness when such agents have been used a supplement of pantothenic acid should be an essential part of the treatment and should be taken routinely for several months afterwards — since these are the times when a deficiency of the vitamin would be most probable. Indeed, following major operations when antibiotics have been used, arthritis has been observed on many occasions.

The neglect of pantothenic acid as an essential factor in human nutrition is all the more surprising when the fact is considered that the vitamin forms an integral part of coenzyme A; a fact that has been known for many years, as well as the other fact that it controls the smooth production of the cortico-steroid hormones in the adrenal cortex.

The author must emphasize here that he in no way holds the opinion that pantothenic acid alone is the be-all and end-all of human or animal nutrition; this would merely be silly and fatuous. All vitamins are equally important in the complex chain of chemical reactions that take place in our bodies. *It is the quantitative aspect that is all important.* In other words, are we eating sufficient amounts of these substances in our daily diet?

The daily amounts of different vitamins required not only by human beings, but also animals, vary enormously, from 1 microgram of vitamin B_{12} (anti-pernicious anaemia factor) to 30mg of ascorbic acid (vitamin C). These are minimal doses and any excess will do no harm, and in fact can usually only do good. It must be realized that human beings are not simply a lot of robots made on exactly the same pattern; we are individuals and our daily requirements of different foods vary enormously from person to person and change as we get older. The "average man", so often referred to by politicians, statisticians and the medical profession simply does not exist.

Thus, we arrive at the important proposition that *all vitamins are equally important in human nutrition and that the amounts required to maintain health and well-being vary greatly from individual to individual and also change as we get older;* a simple common sense fact that has been entirely ignored by statisticians and the medical profession. After all, the strength of a chain depends upon its weakest link and the same applies to the complex chain of metabolic reactions that take place in our bodies. Unfortunately, at the present time one of the weakest links in this metabolic chain is pantothenic acid.

Roger Williams has pointed out: "There is little chance of a spontaneous pantothenic acid deficiency in the human diet because of the widespread distribution of this factor in natural foods." This is an important statement because it once more emphasizes the quantitative aspect of the matter, and undoubtedly this vitamin is required by human beings in comparatively large amounts; at least 25-50mg daily. Compare these figures with the average daily intake of pantothenic acid in the ordinary American diet: 4.5mg/2,500 calories.

That pantothenic acid is required in relatively large amounts in human diets has been shown by Williams. For example, the ratio of pantothenic acid to thiamine (vitamin B_1) in human milk is 18 to 1. It follows, therefore, that human infants need approximately 18 times as much pantothenic acid as thiamine in their diet. Williams has also given figures for the pantothenic acid/thiamine ratios for human and various animal muscles. Muscle is the most abundant tissue in our bodies, as well as animal bodies, and it was found by Williams that human muscle contains 11 times as much pantothenic acid as thiamine; a value nearly twice as much as in other animal muscle tissues, and in the case of pork 11 times as much. The whole of this pantothenic acid must be supplied by the food we eat, since only a small amount is synthesized in the intestinal tract by bacteria, except in the case of vegetarians.

Another important symptom of inadequate supplies of pantothenic acid in the human diet is the so-called "burning feet" syndrome. This is a particularly painful disease and it has been found that injections of 20-40mg of calcium pantothenate daily will cure it.

Nevertheless, it was some far-reaching experiments carried out in the Iowa State Reformatory, U.S.A. that showed beyond all shadow of doubt that pantothenic acid is an essential factor in human nutrition.

This experiment was performed on "volunteers", whose ages varied from 27 to 32. They were fed a complete diet with a calorific value of 3,000, supplemented by the vitamins: thiamine, riboflavin, niacinamide, pyridoxine (vitamin B_6), ascorbic acid (vitamin C), vitamin A and vitamin D, but *no* pantothenic acid.

Analysis of the men's urine showed a decrease in adrenal hormones, which continued to fall progressively during the course of the experiment. The patients became extremely quarrelsome and were easily roused to anger on the slightest pretext. They had dizzy fits and found it difficult to stand erect. If they exerted themselves in any way there was a rapid rise in their pulse rate and they also suffered from respiratory infections, such as sore throats. They readily tired, showed symptoms of muscle weakness, suffered from sleeplessness, stomach upsets and constipation. In 25 days the patients become so seriously ill that the experiment was abruptly stopped, because the investigators feared that permanent damage might occur. Their fears were well founded, because it required a daily dose of 4.0 grams (1/7th of an ounce) of calcium pantothenate plus 25-125mg of cortisone for the first 6 days and then 2.0g of calcium pantothenate for the following 29 days before the men were fully recovered.

This experiment was carried out on normal healthy men, presumably not suffering from stress, yet the symptoms they developed were all typical of adrenal exhaustion and recovery was slow and brought about by what can only be described as massive doses of calcium pantothenate.

Pantothenic Acid and its Relationship to Arthritis

It was found by Dr. W. A. Elliott and the author that the blood pantothenic acid content of persons suffering from rheumatoid arthritis was significantly lower than individuals eating a normal balanced diet, and the greater the severity of the symptoms, the lower was the pantothenic acid content of the blood. Normal people were found to have about 50% more pantothenic acid in the blood than arthritics. Patients with less than half the normal pantothenic acid of blood were completely bedridden and severely crippled. When the pantothenic acid content of the blood of vegetarians (not vegans) was estimated, the value was found to be more than twice that of persons eating a normal meat diet. It was found, however, that vegetarians suffering from rheumatoid arthritis also have a low blood pantothenic acid content, approximately the same as that of rheumatoid arthritics consuming a normal balanced diet.

Some small scale clinical trials were carried out by Dr. Elliott, who first injected calcium pantothenate into rheumatoid arthritics, but the results were inconclusive. Next, he injected an extract of royal jelly into the same patients and the results were again unsuccessful. The reason royal jelly was injected was because we had heard that it had very remarkable effects in controlling rheumatoid arthritis. It was next decided to inject a mixture of calcium pantothenate and royal jelly when it was found that there was a gradual rise in the blood pantothenic acid level and when the value reached normal levels (110-130mcg/100ml whole blood) in 28 days, there was a marked general improvement in 70% of the patients who showed an increase in mobility. When treatment was discontinued the pantothenic acid blood level gradually fell with reappearance of the symptoms.

It was, however, with vegetarian arthritics that the most remarkable results were achieved. When 18 vegetarian rheumatoid arthritics were injected with a mixture of royal jelly and calcium pantothenate, they *all* showed a rapid disappearance of symptoms in 14 days with increase in the blood pantothenic acid level to 130-160mcg/100 ml of blood. Of these 18 patients, only one, a young woman of 30 years, returned after 15 months; the remainder appeared to be completely cured. This woman patient showed a slight recurrence of symptoms, but after a second course of injections appeared to be completely cured. All this took place 11 years ago.

This communication by Dr. Elliott and myself was published in the *Lancet* and produced just one reply from the medical profession. A Dr. Annand wrote saying that he had found that the oral administration of small amounts of calcium pantothenate to osteoarthritics led to relief of the symptoms, but he confirmed the findings of Dr. Elliott and myself that there was a return of the symptoms if treatment was discontinued. One reason why our communication caused no sort of stir in the medical world may have been because we used royal jelly, which is anathema to the medical practitioner, and little wonder, because of the appalling amount of charlatanism that has been practised with this substance, especially on the Continent, and minute amounts of royal jelly have been sold to a gullible public at outrageous prices and in no circumstances could these tiny quantities benefit anybody.

Quite apart, however, from the prejudice that exists among medical practitioners against royal jelly, there are serious economic reasons against its use on a large scale. It is extremely expensive, approximately £1 a gram, and for therapeutic use at least 0.5-1.0g must be taken daily. Moreover, even if world production of royal jelly were to be pooled there simply would not be sufficient quantities to meet world needs.

For this reason substitutes were sought for royal jelly and one such compound was found. Unfortunately, however, although this substance can be produced very cheaply in the laboratory and appears to have no side reactions, to place it on the market under present Ministry of Health regulations would cost many thousands of pounds. It would also take about ten years to prove its worth, just as in the same way if insulin were to have been discovered today it would be at least 10 years before it would be released for general use; never mind that many thousands of sufferers from diabetes would die prematurely in the meantime. They should be grateful that Whitehall is watching the situation carefully in their interests.

The investigations carried out on rats in the U.S.A., which have already been described above, on the effects of acute pantothenic acid deficiency on these animals leading to the onset of all the symptoms of osteoarthritis, as well as the results obtained by Dr. Annand, suggested to Dr. Elliott and myself that perhaps rheumatoid and osteoarthritis are brought about by some kind of upset of the pantothenic acid metabolism of the body.It was finally found that there is such a derangement of the Krebs cycle, which it will be remembered is controlled by the enzyme coenzyme A, and that pantothenic acid forms an integral part of this important enzyme system, at two different points. It was discovered that in rheumatoid arthritis there is some derangement at the beginning of the cycle, whereas in osteoarthritis there appears to be a very serious derangement in the lower part of the cycle and from the experimental evidence Dr. Elliott and I suggested that these results were because of a failure to form adequate amounts of coenzyme A by the body; possibly because people were eating inadequate amounts of pantothenic acid in their daily diet.

Mention has been made above of some small scale clinical trials carried out by Dr. Elliott on rheumatoid arthritis. It was eventually decided, however, to concentrate on osteoarthritics, mainly because of all the difficulties involved, financial and otherwise, in using royal jelly or its substitute, and also because osteoarthritics were found to respond so readily to intramuscular injections in the buttock of a mixture of calcium pantothenate and the amino acid cysteine. The reason for including cysteine was that this amino acid also forms an integral part of the coenzyme A molecule. Furthermore, as has already been mentioned above, osteoarthritics outnumber rheumatoids by 20 to 1.

A summary of some results obtained by a Practitioner in the North of England and who wishes to remain anonymous, and who has treated many hundreds of osteoarthritics with great success, is as follows:-

The dose given was one ampoule of calcium pantothenate (50 mg) and cysteine (15 mg) in 2 cc's water per injection and each patient was initially given 3 injections in 10 days followed by 1 injection per week for 6 weeks.

The patients consisted of the following:—

6 with O.A. of knees

3 with O.A. of lumbar spine

1 with O.A. of knees, hands and wrists

34 cases of O.A. of hip joints which can further be subdivided into 10 early cases, 10 moderate cases and 14 advanced cases — all 44 patients had radiological evidence of osteroarthritis in the joints concerned.

There was a very marked improvement in all patients, shown by increased movement and freedom from pain in the affected joints with the exception of 6 advanced cases in the hip and 1 patient in the knees. Apart from the advanced cases in the hip all patients were asked not to take analgesics and none were prescribed during their six weeks treatment. These patients were all treated between October 1968 and June 1969, and with the exception of 4 of the advanced hip patients all have been followed up to date.

In the light of further experience, the method of treatment has been slightly modified by increasing the quantity of calcium pantothenate to 200mg and the cysteine to 30mg per injection and carrying out the treatment in the following way:

1.   The patient is treated for the first two weeks with three injections per week, say Monday, Wednesday and Friday, i.e. six injections in all.

2.   For the second two weeks, the number of injections is reduced to two a week, say Monday and Friday, i.e., four injections in all.

3.   The number of injections is now reduced to one a week for 14 to 30 days, depending upon the response of the patient to treatment, and thereafter to once a month, again depending on circumstances.

High doses needed?

It should be mentioned here that oral treatment of either rheumatoid or osteoarthritis has given very variable results, but it is felt that a correct dietary approach involving use of polyunsaturated oils (sunflower or safflowerseed oil) coupled with a dietary supplement rich in calcium pantothenate could lead to many patients being relieved without recourse to injections. In the light of the Iowa experiment described above, it is now the author's opinion that the dosage orally administered up to now is far too low. It will be recalled that in the Iowa experiment, the patients required 4g of calcium pantothenate plus varying amounts of cortisone for the first six days after the experiment was stopped, and then this amount of calcium pantothenate was further reduced to 2g a day. It may well be that if osteroarthritics were first treated orally for, say, a week, with massive doses of calcium pantothenate (ca 4g daily) plus 25-50mg of cortisone, and then the amount reduced to 2g a day, and at the same time omitting the cortisone, better results might be achieved. Calcium pantothenate has no side effects whatsoever and persons have taken as much as 10g a day for six weeks without suffering any ill effects at all.

This is very reminiscent of the early days of treatment of patients suffering from Parkinson's disease with L-DOPA. At first patients were treated with very small amounts of this substance (20-50mg daily) and the results were neither conclusive nor satisfactory. It was not until a Dutch physician took his courage in both hands and administered 16g to a patient that it came to be realised that the doses that had been employed in the past were ludicrously low. A similar situation might obtain in the oral treatment of osteoarthritis with calcium pantothenate.

General Discussion

It has been described above how pantothenic acid plays a vital role in the reproduction of insects and animals. It also forms an integral part of coenzyme A and controls the smooth formation of the cortico-steroid hormones in our adrenal glands. It is claimed here that lack of pantothenic acid, or inadequate amounts of this vitamin in our daily diet, also leads eventually over a long period of years to the onset of rheumatoid or osteoarthritis.

Dr. Roger Williams has offered odds of 10 to 1 that if prospective human mothers were given a daily supply of 50mg of pantothenic acid there would be a substantial decrease in the number and severity of reproductive failures. Complete elimination is not to be expected because of the relationship between genetics and nutrition. There is a close relationship between genes, the carriers of our inheritance factors and many of the enzyme systems in our bodies. Thus, if genes are responsible for the control of the enzyme systems in our bodies, it follows that the enzyme patterns in different people must vary, and as has been pointed out above, each person must be treated as an individual and not as a robot made up on exactly the same pattern as his neighbour.

The author is willing to offer even greater odds than Dr. Williams of a 100 to 1 that if every infant at birth were supplied with 25-50mg of pantothenic acid and continued to consume this amount for the remainder of its life span, and if pregnant women were supplied with at least 50mg of pantothenic acid during pregnancy, many of the ills, physical and mental, from which the human race suffers would be things of the past.

If my interpretation of the data be correct, arthritis must now be added to the list of deficiency diseases caused by consuming inadequate amounts of pantothenic acid in the daily diet. There can never be complete lack of this vitamin in the food we eat, because of its ubiquitous distribution, but on account of its instability to such factors as heat and storage and the advent of processed foods, the world population must generally be consuming inadequate amounts daily.

Arthritis, whether rheumatoid or osteoarthritis, is on the increase the world over. In 1965 there were known to be 10,000,000 arthritics of both kinds in the U.S.A. Today it has risen to 30,000,000. It has always been known to be present on a small scale in the Latin South American countries, but is now rapidly increasing. It is increasing at an alarming rate in the urban districts of Japan, although the disease was practically unknown in that country 40 or 50 years ago. In Great Britain it has increased from 3,000,000 in 1965 to 6,000,000 at the present time and is now on the increase in India.

It may well be asked why there should be this serious increase in arthritis over the past 10 to 15 years. One answer, so far as the author is concerned, is that the world population is eating more and more of the highly processed foods first made so popular in the U.S.A., and this change in eating habits is spreading to other countries, with the exception, perhaps, of India. It is little wonder that these processed foods have gained world wide popularity, because they are very palatable, and what is simpler than to serve up an apparently appetising meal by using a can opener or heating something from the freezer? Whether the contents are nutritious and will maintain the health and well-being of the consumer is quite another matter. It is probable that the population of the U.S.A. is the best fed and worst nourished in the world.

As far as India is concerned there may be another explanation for the sudden increase in arthritis among the population, namely, the failure of the monsoon rain over several years, leading in turn to the failure of the rice crop, which is a staple article of food in the Indian diet. The Indians are now turning to other substitutes for rice, such as ordinary and sweet potatoes, which are poor sources of pantothenic acid, whereas, as has been pointed out above, rice husks are a comparatively rich source of this vitamin.

There was one country in the world where arthritis was

unknown until recently, Greenland, the land of the Eskimos. The Eskimos used to live mainly on a diet of raw seal flesh. When a seal was killed its liver was extracted and then divided up into different sized portions and the largest distributed to the more important members of the tribe, the rest of the flesh was then eaten. Now, however, the Eskimos have taken to eating processed foods, and arthritis is rapidly making its appearance.

Arthritis, of whatever form, is an insidious disease and may take long years before symptoms make their appearance. On the other hand, it is possible that arthritic symptoms make their appearance earlier in some mild or minor forms which have not been recognized by the clinician for what they are. For example, sufferers from what is called "muscular lumbago" as well as other apparently trivial aches and pains, have obtained quick relief when injected with calcium pantothenate and cysteine, and it may well be that these are early signs of the onset of arthritis and should not be neglected.

We are all of us eating some pantothenic acid in our diet; inadequate though these amounts may be. It has already been seen that complete absence of pantothenic acid in the diet can produce sudden and dramatic effects, *vide* the Iowa Prison experiment, but it is the consumption of inadequate amounts of the vitamin over a long number of years that eventually leads to the onset of this crippling disease. If the statement be true that the average daily intake of pantothenic acid per person in the U.S.A. is 4.5mg, is it surprising, if the author's interpretation of the data be correct, that arthritis is rapidly increasing?

The question may well be asked, why is it that, if there is such a serious lack of pantothenic acid in our daily diet today, arthritis is not more widespread and attacking every person consuming such a deficient diet? The answer is that our requirements, not only for pantothenic acid but also other vitamins, varies enormously from individual to individual, and that what may be an inadequate amount for one person is sufficient for another. This is well shown by the outbreaks of scurvy on old sailing ships. For instance, the Portuguese explorer, Vasco de Gama, in his voyage round the Cape of Good Hope to India set sail with a crew of 160 men, but by the time he reached India his crew was reduced to 60, the remainder died of scurvy. Presumably the 60 survivors had required much smaller amounts of ascorbic acid (vitamin C) compared with those that had succumbed and died.

If my interpretation of the data be correct, then it follows that if every individual could be sure of consuming in his or her daily diet at least 25-50mg of pantothenic acid, preferably from early infancy, arthritis would be as rare as other vitamin deficiency diseases such as scurvy, beri-beri, pellagra and rickets.

However, there is this alarming thought that should be borne in mind that arthritis may, in the years to come, prove to be a far greater menace to the human race than other deficiency diseases that have been overcome in the past. Those deficiency diseases, with the exception perhaps of pellagra, which spread from South America across Europe to the Middle East, were mainly confined to particular regions, whereas arthritis is becoming world wide in its incidence, because people are eating more and more of these so-called sophisticated, highly processed, but very palatable foods of low nutritional value lacking health giving vital elements.

Addendum to
'Arthritis, Its cause and control'
by Dr. R. J. Woodward, 1981

Soon after writing this little book in 1975 Dr. Eustace Barton-Wright died and I have often wondered what he would have said about the current state of knowledge of the arthritic diseases and the continuing scepticism of the medical profession about his vitamin deficiency theory.

I knew Dr. Barton-Wright well in the last few years of his life — we were both convinced of the value of alternative medical therapies despite our scientific backgrounds rooted in biochemistry, pharmacy, organic and analytical chemistry. The pantothenic acid theory seemed sound and I became converted to a belief in Barton-Wright's concept but always advocated that dietary and lifestyle changes should also be adopted by patients because the long term effects of pantothenic acid deficiencies seemed bound to embrace more problems than just arthritis and rheumatism those diseases being merely the readily recognisable manifestation of a deficiency state. Depression, allergies, including those to food and the environment, general weakness, susceptibility to infection and failure to overcome stress are also allied to the metabolic disorders caused by long term pantothenic acid deficiency.

In the years since Dr. Barton-Wright's death we have seen virtually no progress in the conventional medical treatment of arthritis. New drugs abound but are as **fundamentally useless** as those used before. Surgery now covers more joints than it did but this is not indicative of progress in finding the fundamental cause of arthritis! In the alternative medical field we have seen the rise of Devil's Claw, a herbal treatment which has not proved a great success because its promoters treated it like a drug and looked for active principles and all that nonsense. As a whole herb it may have helped people because, being a plant, it has a store of nutrients which include traces of vitamins — even pantothenic acid! Considerable public relations effort has been used to promote the herb but the authorities failed to recognise it as being of any benefit.

Another product in the alternative medical field which has received much public relations effort from the main world producer has been the Green Lipped Mussel Extract. This has been banned in many countries. Again the promoters have made the error of treating the product as if it was a drug and a 'cure'. It has a vast spectrum of ingredients and scientists have tried to find an active principle without success. This extract could be of value as a dietary supplement because of its comprehensive contents but one wonders what more it has to offer than ordinary seaweed tablets combined with a wholesome diet including shellfish! Clinical trials of the substance are currently continuing but I see nothing yet which is likely to change the Government's view that the green lipped mussel cannot be recommended for arthritis and rheumatism.

Pantothenic acid has been subjected to one clinical trial since Dr. Barton-Wright's death and the results were published in The Practitioner (Practitioner, February 1980, volume 224, pages 208-211). The results were inconclusive but the authors felt more research was indicated particularly as regards the use in rheumatoid arthritis. No-one has been willing to undertake further research because there is no monopoly market to be exploited. Pantothenic acid (or calcium pantothenate) cannot be patented like drugs. I conclude that the present situation is much as it was in 1975 when Dr. Barton-Wright wrote this book.

The pantothenic acid treatment for arthritis and rheumatism remains. The recommended products:—

Osteo-arthritis:— Injections of calcium pantothenate and cysteine.

Rheumatoid Arthritis:— Capsules of calcium pantothenate, cysteine and unsaturated fatty acid.

The use of calcium pantothenate as a dietary supplement 3 x 50mg daily as a preventive is recommended, ideally with a natural style of diet.

As a control for sufferers there is no maximum amount recommended because years of deficiency will have caused many enzyme pathway distortions and in order to get the right pathway established once more could take a long time. However, two to thirty grammes a day have been used either as a powder or high strength 500mg tablets. The usual amounts are 6 to 10 500mg tablets daily at meals.

Dietary control in general should always be considered and a natural style of diet or even one with more restrictions such as the "Original Cantassium Dietary System" may be adopted. Increasing the ratio of polyunsaturated fats to saturated fats in the diet can also be helpful using sunflower oil, safflower oil, evening primrose oil and fish liver oils as supplements or in cooking.

Appendix

Useful Addresses

Natural Diets,

The Cantassium Co.
225 Putney Bridge Road,
London SW15 2PY.

Injections of Calcium Pantothenate and Information,

Koch Light Laboratories,
Colnbrook,
Buckinghamshire.

The Cantassium Co.
225 Putney Bridge Road,
London SW15 2PY.

Natural Therapies,

The Nature Cure Clinic.
Oldbury Place,
London, SW1.

The Kent Private Clinic.
Sandwich,
Kent.

The Homoeopathic and Osteopathic Clinic.
29 Upper Lattimore Road,
St. Albans,
Hertfordshire.

Pantothenic Acid content of foods (in mg) per 100g (approx. 4 oz.)

Food	Pantothenic Acid (mg)
Wholemeal Bread	0.7
Wholewheat Flour	1.5
Raw Oatmeal	1.0
Cheddar Cheese	0.3
Milk, dried, skimmed	3.5
Egg yolk, (raw)	3.5
Liver, lamb's, (raw)	7.0
Chicken, breast, (raw)	0.7
Chicken, leg (raw)	1.0
Beef, (raw)	0.4
Salmon, canned	0.50
Sardines, canned in oil	0.50
Shrimps, cooked	0.30
Apricots, fresh, (raw)	0.30
Apricots, dried, (raw)	0.70
Bananas, (raw)	0.20
Dates, dried	0.80
Grapefruit, (raw)	0.23

Melon, (raw)	0.25
Oranges or orange juice, (fresh)	0.15
Prunes, dried, (raw)	0.35
Raspberries, (raw)	0.20
Beans, broad, (raw)	5.4
Beetroot, (raw)	0.12
Broccoli tops, (raw)	1.0
Brussels sprouts, (raw)	0.40
Carrots, (raw)	0.25
Cauliflower, (raw)	0.60
Celery, (raw)	0.40
Cucumber, (raw)	0.30
Kale, (raw)	0.30
Mushrooms, (raw)	2.0
Parsnips, (raw)	0.50
Peas, (raw)	1.5
Tomatoes, canned	0.2
Watercress	0.10
Peanuts, (raw)	2.7

(Chart prepared from The Composition of Foods by
R. A. McCance & E. M. Widdowson)

GENERAL DIET ADVICE

Everyone should be aware of the dangers of the modern diet. With our shops and supermarkets crammed with appetizing looking processed food and convenience foods now being the norm, it is all too easy to find oneself wooed by such fare into a state of poor nutrition.

Here are the main diet dangers:-

FIBRE — too little

Refined flours are often low in fibre. Valuable fibre can be lost from fruit and vegetables by peeling and discarding skins, etc. Bake or boil potatoes in their "jackets" and eat both flesh and skins. Use a cereal bran regularly in baking, etc. Eat nuts and dried fruit for snacks. 100% wholewheat flour can be used for home-baked bread and baking.

FAT — too much

Many of the population consume too much fat, particularly cholesterol/saturated fat. It is not uncommon to find people on diets where 50% of the food consumed daily is in the form of fat. The way to reduce this to a more sensible proportion of about 20% to 25% is to grill food instead of frying, to use the less fatty types of meat such as chicken, and to avoid the lavish use of butter, margarine and cream.

SUGAR — too much

Avoid over-use of this refined carbohydrate by not taking it in drinks such as tea and coffee, by eating fresh fruit instead of syrupy canned fruit and by getting out of the habit of eating sweets and chocolates and sugary snacks.

SALT — too much

Use salt only sparingly at table and in cooking. Avoid salty snacks such as salted nuts and crisps. Other items which are highly salted are yeast extracts, savoury spreads, smoked fish and bacon. They should be avoided or eaten in moderation.

PROCESSED FOODS — too much

Fresh fruit and vegetables are best for your health. Avoid the freezer cabinet and the junk-food shelves in the shops. Eat wholewheat bread instead of white. Keep out of the bakers and bake your own items using 100% wholewheat flour.

ALCOHOL — too much

Too much alcohol can lead to addiction. Spirits should be largely avoided in favour of wines and beers, but always in moderation.

SUGGESTED DIET BALANCE

45% fresh fruit and vegetables
15% bakery items
20% fats, oils, nuts and seeds
20% meat, fish, eggs and dairy produce

Every day eat at least 1 large helping of fresh green leafy vegetables and 1 large mixed salad. Two of the daily meals should contain a reasonable helping of protein — meat, fish or eggs. Up to 6 slices of wholewheat bread (preferably home-baked) can be eaten. Regarding fats and oils, a soft margarine high in polyunsaturates and the use of sunflower, safflower and soya oil for cooking and salad oil would be wise. As already discussed, sparing use of salt and sugar, constant use of fresh foods instead of processed and convenience foods, plenty of cereal fibre and minimal alcohol.

"Governments and food producers should encourage the eating of foods that are closer to their natural state than are the refined items that reach the average British meal table."

Royal College of Physicians, 1980

Bear in mind that processing of food by cooking, canning, may destroy from 20% to 50% of the Pantothenic Acid in food. Some foods, although they have a reasonable Pantothenic Acid content, are only eaten in small amounts, e.g. broad beans. Others, with a lower content, can be eaten in more substantial amounts, e.g. wholewheat bread.

It is possible to enjoy a meal or snack comprising several items which contain Pantothenic Acid. (Two slices of wholewheat bread, 1 oz cheddar cheese, 1 oz watercress followed by 1 oz raw peanuts or 1 oz dried (raw) apricots should contain about 4mg Pantothenic Acid. 4 oz lamb's liver, 3 oz cauliflower, 2 oz mushrooms and 3 oz potatoes contain over 5 mg Pantothenic Acid.)

USEFUL RECIPES

WINTER SALAD — serves 2

1 oz (25 g) of each of the following:
raw Brussels sprouts, prepared
raw grated carrot
raw cauliflower, chopped small
raw parsnip
fresh peanuts
raw mushroom, sliced

Combine in a salad bowl and dress with oil/vinegar dressing and season to taste.

Whole salad gives about 1.5 mg Pantothenic Acid.

SUMMER SALAD 1   — serves 1

1 oz raw broad beans, chopped small or sliced (25 g)
3 lettuce leaves torn into pieces
2 spring onions, prepared and sliced
1 oz raw mushrooms

Combine in a salad bowl and dress with oil/vinegar dressing and season to taste.

Whole salad gives just over 2 mg Pantothenic Acid.

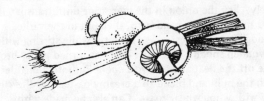

SUMMER SALAD 2 — serves 1

1 oz (25 g) each of the following prepared vegetables:

sliced cucumber, chopped celery, raw sliced mushrooms, grated carrot and raw peas.

Combine in a salad bowl and dress with oil/lemon juice dressing and season to taste. 3 or 4 pinches of sugar can also be sprinkled over, if desired.

Gives just over 1 mg Pantothenic Acid.

LIVER PATÉ – 4 servings

8 oz lambs' liver (250 g)
1 small onion, peeled and chopped
1 oz soft margarine (25 g)
1 sage leaf, finely chopped or 2 pinches dried thyme
1 small clove garlic, peeled

salt and freshly ground black pepper
1 heaped tablespoon dried, skimmed milk,
    reconstituted with 2 tablespoons water

Cut out and discard strings etc. from the liver and chop
finely. Fry the onion in the margarine until transparent.
Add the liver pieces and herb, then put in the garlic,
through a garlic press. Heat through while stirring with
a wooden spoon. When the liver has turned pinky-brown
take off the heat and allow to cool. Put into a blender
with the milk and blend to a creamy paste. Eat the same
day with wholewheat toast. Can also be made with
chicken livers. (Add a little more milk to blender if
mixture is too dry to blend.)

Each of 4 servings on wholewheat toast gives about 2 mg
Pantothenic Acid.

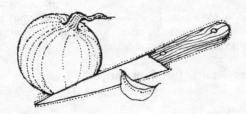

FRUIT CRUMBLE — 4 servings

This is served hot or cold and can have a base of any kind
of stewed, sweetened fruit in season — apple, apricot, plum
etc., or any combination. You will need about 1 lb fruit.

Topping:
4 oz wholewheat flour (100 g)
1 heaped teaspoon wheat bran
2 heaped teaspoons sesame seeds
2 heaped teaspoons sunflower seeds
1 heaped teaspoon brown sugar

Rub in the flour, margarine and bran. Use a fork to mix the
seeds and sugar into the bowl. The topping is now ready to
sprinkle over the prepared fruit which should be put into a
Pyrex or similar ovenprooof dish. Bake for 10 to 12 minutes
on the top shelf of a preheated oven at Regulo 8 (450°F or
232°C). The fruit should be slightly tart.

Gives less than 0.5 mg Pantothenic Acid per portion but is
high in fibre.

MUSHROOM QUICHE — 4 servings

Pastry:
4 oz plain wholewheat flour (100 g)
2 oz soft margarine (50 g)
cold water

Put the flour into a large bowl with the margarine.
Blend with a fork and then rub in with the fingers
until the mixture resembles fine breadcrumbs. Put
in enough cold water to bind into one soft ball of

dough. Use more flour to roll out. Lift half the
pastry and slip the rolling pin underneath. Lift on
to the quiche dish (a medium sized one) and carefully remove the rolling pin. Press the pastry into
the dish and trim off excess with a knife. Now
pull the pastry slightly out over the edge of the dish.
Prick the bottom lightly with a fork to release air
during baking. Put on to a baking sheet and bake
on the top shelf of the oven (preheated) at Regulo 7
(425°F or 218°C) for 12 to 15 minutes. While you
are waiting for the case to bake, prepare the filling.

Filling:
2 eggs
½ pint milk (275 ml) made from dried skimmed milk
    reconstituted using double the amount of granules
4 oz mushrooms, washed and finely chopped

Lightly whisk the eggs and milk. Pour into the cooked
pastry case. Sprinkle in the chopped mushrooms. Put
carefully back into the oven, still in the quiche dish,and
bake on a lower heat at Regulo 5 (375°F or 190°C) for
about 35 to 40 minutes until set. Use a shelf just above
centre of the oven. Sprinkle with a little chopped parsley
just before serving. Serve hot or cold.

Gives just over 1 mg of Pantothenic Acid per portion.

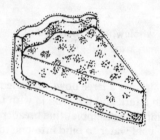